FulFUELING

Are you fueling your body properly?

1st Edition

By
Alex Coffey

www.fastfit60.com

Introduction

The low-fat craze of the 1990s was a dismal failure. Not only did few people lose weight and keep it off, but many more became addicted to the sugar that was used to replace the fat in most manufactured "low-fat" foods. This caused an effect opposite of the intended one. Many people gained weight—and those who did manage to lose weight at the time gained it back and weighed more than they had weighed before going on a low-fat "diet".

Furthermore, you may be eating more sugar than you think. Sugar is often added to pre-packaged food without the average consumer being aware of it. Terms like "high fructose corn syrup" "maltose" and "dextrose"—along with about 50 others—make it easy for manufacturers to "hide" sugar. They also make it easy for consumers to overindulge without even knowing it. By cooking your own food using real ingredients with recognizable names, you can easily take control of what you are eating.

So, if low-fat isn't the ideal option for healthy eating, what is?

The answer is a diet low in carbs and high in fat made of real food.

- It doesn't have to be restrictive.
- It doesn't have to be difficult.
- You don't have to feel hungry.
- It can be easy and it can be delicious.

By preparing and eating the foods in this book, you will lose weight and feel better doing it.

Contents

Dinner

Lunch

Breakfast

Snacks

Treat Day

Everyone loves when the day comes to have their cheat meal. We look forward to those times when you gather for a meal, laughing creating memories together. Having a cheat day every week allows you to indulge and eat the things that you really love especially those that are rich, sweet and very much tasty. These may include a slice of cake, burgers, pizzas, chocolates, ice cream – pretty much everything that you don't normally eat when you are on a diet. As for me I consider my cheat food to be ice cream. Aside from satisfying my sweet tooth craving, I get to eat it with my whole family, brothers, sisters, nephews and nieces – it's a great way to connect with your loved ones while celebrating meeting your commitment to being fit.

I believe we all have funny stories that involve food and family. Every time I have my favorite treat I am reminded of "our ice cream journey". One day my older brother, twin brother and I had the biggest craving for ice cream. Not just any kind of ice cream. No… We had the biggest craving for gelato ice cream! For those of you that are unfamiliar with this amazing treat, it is a different form of ice cream that has more milk than cream and denser that the usual ice cream making it yummier. So now you know ice cream is my kryptonite and the one food I cannot give up.

Moving along with my story, it was a random Saturday night and we were on a late night hunt to find our gelatos ice cream. What should have been a simple trip to the ice cream store turned into one of the funniest nights we have had in a long time. I will spare the details and share the highlights. Unfortunately, the store up the street from us where we always go to was closed. So, like anyone on a mission, a mission to satisfy our sweet tooth no less, our hunt began. We were not going home until we had gelato.

We looked up store after store, rushing to the next one open, but they kept closing before we were able to get there or showing up in the GPS as closed already. But we were persistent and we continued our mission to satisfy that craving, we finally found a gelato store that was open. Whew! Thank goodness! We set the GPS and we were on our way.

We joked and laughed together the entire way. Then as we approached the ice cream store we noticed that the area was a lot busier than the usual. We slowly approached a parking spot close to a nearby intersection and suddenly heard a loud bang. To our surprise, somebody stopped her car in the middle of the intersection! She then put her car in reverse and began backing up quickly in an attempt to park in the spot that we were pulling

pulling in and sure enough, she hit us.

We got out of the car, asked the young lady what happened and why she decided to back up in the middle of the intersection. Her response was so puzzling I couldn't help but smile. Her excuse for hitting us was she had never been so excited to see a parking spot. So without thinking or looking,
she immediately reversed her car.

After we had that situation handled we decided we were walking to the gelato store. I placed my order last and as I look down, I see my two brothers each eating a pint size ice cream. They read my mind, "go big or go home." Imagine three guys walking down the sidewalk on a Saturday night all eating three separate tubs of ice cream.

Why am I sharing this with you? As you can see I'm not all fitness and I love that my ice cream cheat day can became an adventure. It's so important to have fun and BE ALIVE! Do things that make you happy. Let's face it we are only human and enjoying life is part of living a healthier life. Overall, this will be helpful in realizing your goal.

I want you to know that we all need a cheat meal to not only reset our metabolisms but to satisfy our cravings. I would like to share why a cheat day, or meal, is important in your fitness journey. One of the greatest benefits is feeling satisfied. Could you imagine the smiles on our faces when we finally got that big tub of gelato? I felt like a big kid! To have that discipline all week, reward myself with my favorite treat and to have that wonderful feeling of gratification as we walked away, it was awesome.
I am certain you have had that same feeling at some point. Imagine having it every week.

An addition I find cheat day helps you avoid redundancy and boredom. When people eat the same thing over and over again, they tend to become 'fed up' and sometimes just give up. The craving becomes powerful and eventually some just give in. I have also found it's important we are not only physically fit but we also have to make sure that our emotional well-being
is stable and strong.

Many people have found that having the autonomy to treat themselves is key to keeping that emotional balance and avoid burn out. Let's face it, everyone likes to be rewarded, especially when they did a good job. Punishing yourself by being too strict isn't healthy or something that can be maintained over time. I find rewarding yourself once in a while boosts morale and makes you want to push harder to improve yourself.

The last benefit I want to mention is adding those extra nutrients that our body needs. As I've mentioned, aside from re-setting our metabolism, it also allow us to add more nutrients in the body. Remember that if you are following a strict diet, there are some nutrients that are not enough like a good amount of protein or carbohydrates. Eating lean red meat has more proteins than a simple baked fish or grilled chicken. So it's good to have a cheat day once in a while as long as you don't go overboard or overdo it.

A word of caution however, cheat meals can sometimes become a mission to overindulge, eating everything you want versus just making sure you get that one thing you MUST HAVE. I encourage you to have your treats inmoderation and take your overall goals into consideration when having your own cheat day. Be realistic and still plan your meals well. Don't let this be an excuse to eat as many ice cream or as many burgers and fries as you can. As much as possible, if you can, try to still avoid eating pro-cessed foods. This will not only ruin your diet but bad for your health as well. Let me again remind you that overindulgence has its consequences. Too muchof anything is bad for a person, eating is no exception.

Overall, cheat days are not really bad as long as you still practice eating smart and have control and discipline for yourself. Don't look at cheat days as burden. Learn to relax, have fun and enjoy the day! Live a little, love more, laugh and enjoy life!

Now that we are done talking about the fun part, let's move on and be serious with our discipline.in
and sure enough, she hit us.

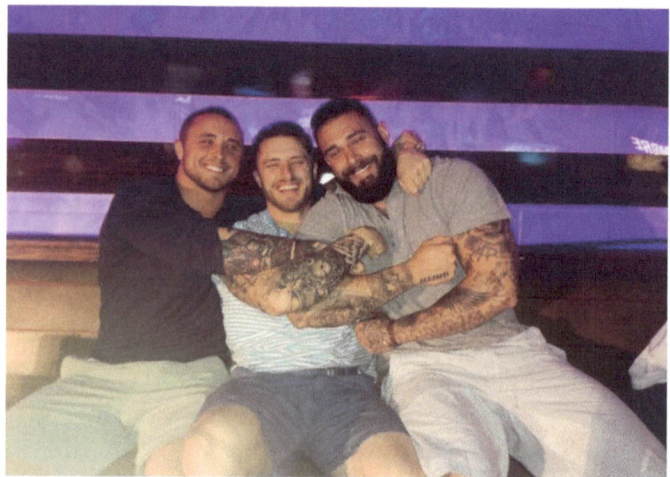

DINNER

Dinner

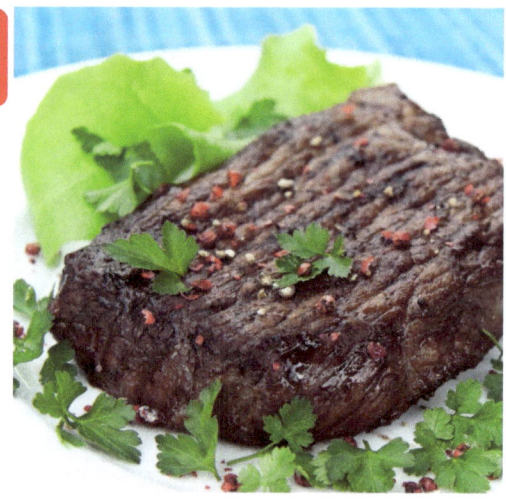

Roast Bison

Ingredients:
- 2 tbsp olive oil
- 1 3-pound boneless bison roast
- 1 cup yellow onion roughly chopped
- 2 cup baby carrots
- 2 cups red potatoes sliced or roughly diced
- 2 cups chicken or vegetable stock
- 1 ½ tsp Himalayan or sea salt to taste
- ½ tsp freshly ground black pepper

Directions:
1. Heat olive oil in a skillet over high heat. Add onions and brown them lightly.
2. Sprinkle bison with salt and pepper. Place roast in a slow cooker on high heat. Add stock and 1 cup of water. Add onions. Cook on high for 5 hours.
3. Add vegetables and cook for 3 hours on low or until done.

Nutritional Information:
8 servings

Calories: 176
Protein: 7.2
Carbohydrate: 11
Fat: 8.4

Tips:
Choose grass-fed bison
Shoulder and rump are best, but chuck or round steak are also options

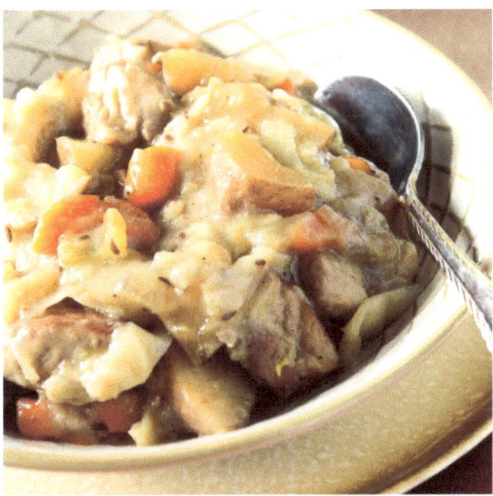

Dinner

Chicken Slow Cooked with Cabbage and Carrots

Ingredients:
- 1 ½ cups onion sliced vertically or roughly chopped
- 2 tsp olive oil
- 2 cups baby carrots
- 2 cups red potatoes cut into fourths
- 1 cup chicken broth
- 1 tsp minced garlic
- ¾ tsp Himalayan or seas salt
- ½ tsp freshly ground pepper
- 1 tsp oregano
- 6 bone in chicken thighs or 9 legs

Directions:
1. Use half of the olive oil to coat the slow cooker. Add onions and top with carrots and potatoes. Add broth.
2. Cover the chicken evenly with a mixture of the seasonings.
3. Heat remaining oil in a skillet and brown chicken about 3 minutes on each side.
4. Add chicken on top of the vegetable in the slow cooker. Cook on low for about 3 ½ hours or until chicken is done.

Nutritional Information:
6 servings
Calories: 285
Protein: 23
Carbohydrate: 15
Fat: 14

Tips:
Use low sodium chicken broth. Add Himalayan or sea salt for flavor enhancement. This allows the cook to control how much sodium is used, as well as incorporates a healthier option than most full-sodium broths use.

Dinner

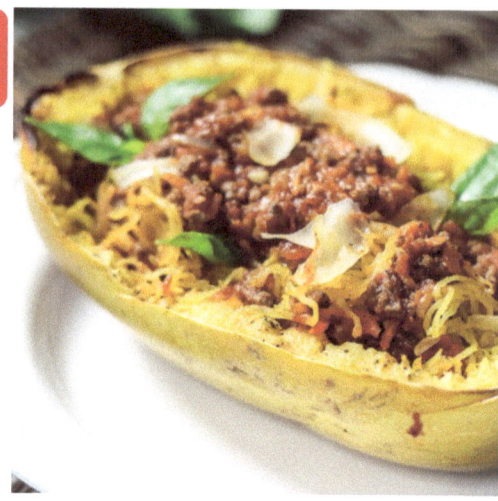

Roasted Sphaghetti Squash and Almonds

Ingredients:
- 1 spaghetti squash
- 1 head of garlic
- 1 tbsp olive oil
- 2 tbsp almonds sliced
- 2 cups zucchini diced
- 4 ounces cheddar cheese

Directions:
1. Preheat oven to 350-degrees F
2. Split the spaghetti squash in half and scoop out the seeds. Place both halves face up on a baking sheet.
3. Clean and slice the garlic. Add to the interior of the two squash halves. Add oil, almonds, and lastly zucchini.
4. Place the baking sheet on the upper rack and cook for 30-40 minutes or until the squash easily separates from the skin.
5. Remove from oven and cool in the refrigerator for at least 20 before separating the squash from the skin.
6. Remove interior with a fork and serve. Pour melted cheese over individual servings.

Nutritional Information:
6 servings
Calories: 204
Protein: 6.6
Carbohydrate: 13
Fat: 15

Tips:
Spaghetti squash can easily be used as a "low carb" "go to" substitute for pasta in any Italian dish. Cover it in marinara sauce or even Alfredo. Add meatballs or more vegetables.

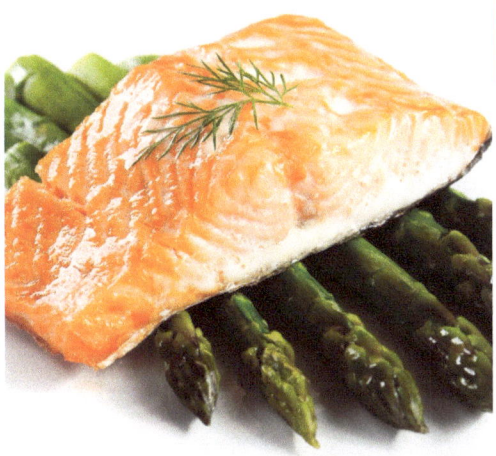

Dinner

Grilled Salmon and Asparagus

Ingredients:
- 3 pounds salmon fillets with the skin
- 2 tbsp olive oil
- 2 tsp low sodium soy sauce
- 1tsp garlic powder
- 1 tsp lemon pepper
- 2 pounds asparagus, trimmed
- 1 tbsp garlic minced
- Himalayan or sea salt
- Freshly ground black pepper

Directions:
1. Coat salmon with oil. Coat grill with oil and heat to medium.
2. Mix soy sauce, garlic powder, and lemon pepper. Brush over salmon. Place fillets on grill skin side up to get sear marks. Gently flip over and cook skin side down over lower heat until done. Remove.
3. Trim asparagus. Toss with garlic, salt, and pepper. Place in an oiled pan on grill for about 5 minutes or until done.

Nutritional Information:
6 servings
Calories: 222
Protein: 11
Carbohydrate: 35.6
Fat: 16

Tips:
Eat salmon regularly. As a fatty fish, it has been shown to improve mood and overall health

Dinner

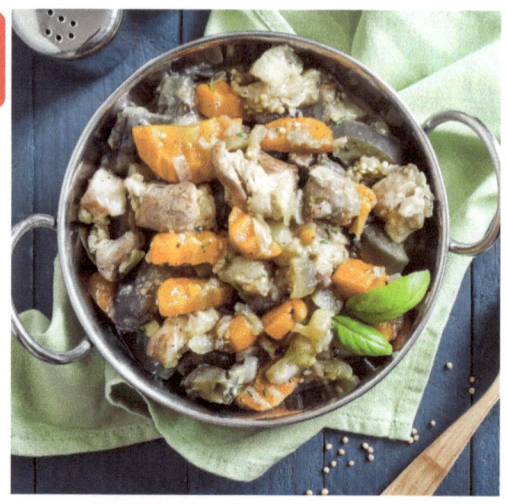

Beef and Vegetable Stew

Ingredients:
- 2 pounds beef stew meat cut into 1-inch cubes
- ½ tsp Himalayan or sea salt
- ½ tsp freshly ground pepper
- ½ cup yellow or white onion sliced or rough cut
- 3 cups red potatoes
- 4 carrots sliced
- 2 stalks of celery sliced
- 1 ½ cups of beef broth
- 1 tsp garlic powder
- 1 tsp paprika

Directions:
1. Combine all ingredients into a slow cooker.
2. Cover and cook on low for 10-12 hours or high for 4-6

Nutritional Information:
6 servings
Calories: 329
Protein: 34
Carbohydrate: 15
Fat: 10

Tips:
One pound of potatoes equals about seven to nine small red potatoes and yields about three cups sliced or rough-cut.

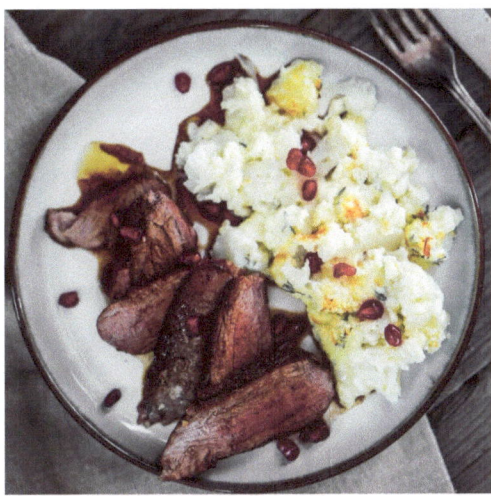

Dinner

Steak and Mashed Cauliflower

Ingredients:
- 4 8-ounce, 1 1/3-inch thick steak fillets
- 1 tsp coriander seeds
- 2 tsp freshly ground black pepper
- 2 tsp olive oil
- 1 head cauliflower cut into florettes
- 1 tsp Himalayan or sea salt
- butter or grated cheese as desired

Directions:
1. Mix the coriander seeds and half of the pepper. Dry rub the steak fillets with the mixture. Use 1 tbsp oil to grease a large skillet and place on medium heat. Add the fillet when the skillet is warm.
2. Turn the steaks periodically and remove when it feels correct to the touch. Rare is soft, well done is firmer.
3. Let it set for 5 minutes to redistribute the juices.
4. In a large pot, bring water to boil. Add cauliflower and cook 10 minutes or until tender. Loosely drain. Mix with a mixer or in a food processor. Add remaining oil and mix until smooth. Season with remaining pepper and salt.
5. Serve with steak. Add butter or cheese if desired.

Nutritional Information:
4 servings
Calories: 423
Protein: 51
Carbohydrate: 2
Fat: 23

Tips:
When cooking 1 1/3-inch steak on medium temperature, follow this guide:
Rare: About 2¼ minutes each side
Medium-rare: About 3¼ minutes each side
Medium: About 4½ minutes each side
Well: About 51/2 minutes each side

Dinner

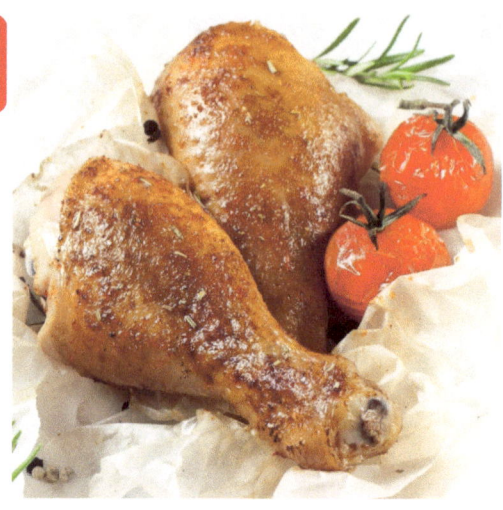

Roasted Turkey Drums

Ingredients:
- 4 turkey legs
- Himalayan or sea salt
- Freshly ground pepper
- Real butter- preferably stick butter for ease of use

Directions:
1. Preheat oven to 350-degree F
2. Rinse turkey legs and pat dry.
3. Spread butter evenly over the legs. Sprinkle salt and pepper over them evenly.
4. Lay the legs on a wire rack placed over a pan in the oven. The pan collects drippings as the legs roast.
5. Cook to 45 minutes. Turn the legs and cook the other side for 45 minutes.
6. Remove from the oven and let sit for 10 minutes to cool and redistribute the juices.

Nutritional Information:
4 servings
Calories: 399
Protein: 39.8
Carbohydrate:
Fat: 24.3

Tips:
Using a meat thermometer takes the guesswork out of thoroughly cooking meat. The center of a turkey drumstick should be 180-degrees F.

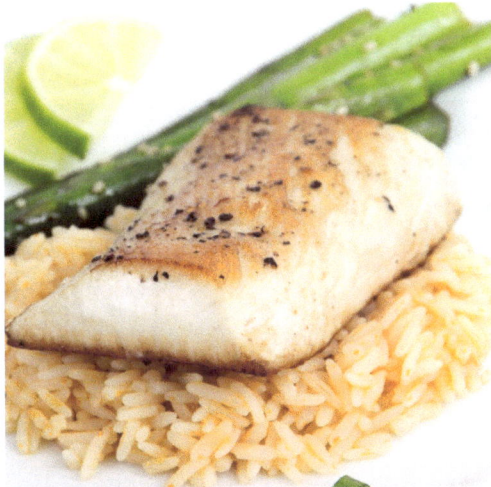

Dinner

Mahi Mahi with Rice

Ingredients:
- 2 ⊠pounds Mahi-Mahi (about 4 fillets)
- 2 tbsp fresh lemon juice
- ¼ tsp garlic salt
- ¼ ⊠tsp freshly ground black pepper
- 1 cup mayonnaise
- ¼ cup onion white or yellow, diced
- 4 cups water
- I package boil in bag rice

Directions:
1. Preheat oven to 425-degrees F
2. Rinse fish. Place in oven safe baking dish and add lemon, garlic salt, and pepper.
3. Mix mayonnaise and onions. Spread over fish.
4. Bake for 25 minutes
5. Boil 4 cups of water in a medium pot and drop in one unopened bag of rice. Boil uncovered for 10-12 minutes. Remove and drain.
6. Cut open and serve with fish. Add vegetables if desired.

Nutritional Information:
4 servings
Calories: 672
Protein: 213
Carbohydrate: 1.1
Fat: 44

Tips:
To avoid sticky rice, fluff with a fork before serving. Add butter if desired.

Dinner

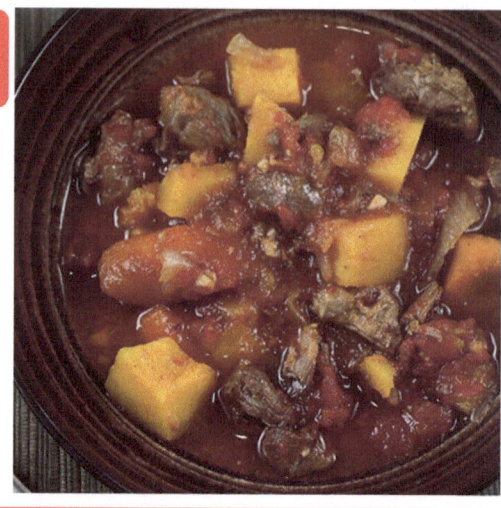

Lamb and Beef Stew

Ingredients:
- 2 tbsp olive oil
- 1 pound lamb stew meat or shoulder cut into 1-inch cubes
- ½ cup onion finely chopped (about 1 medium peeled)
- 12 cups low sodium beef broth
- 4 cups beets peeled and diced (about 3 medium) reserve the greens
- ½ medium head of cabbage shredded (about 1 ¼ pounds)
- 2 cups tomatoes diced (about 3 medium tomatoes)
- 2 stalks celery diced
- ½ cup carrots chopped
- ½ tsp freshly ground pepper
- 1 pint sour cream

Directions:
1. Heat oil over medium heat in a large pot until it is hot. Add the lamb to brown it. Stir in the onion and cook for about 2 minutes.
2. Add broth, beets, cabbage, tomatoes, carrots, and pepper. Bring to a boil. Reduce heat to medium-low and cover. Simmer for about 2 hours.
3. Add celery and chopped beet greens. Simmer for 15-30 minutes. Season to taste. Serve with a dollop of sour cream.

Nutritional Information:
8 servings
Calories: 239
Protein: 16
Carbohydrate: 7.6
Fat: 9

Tips:
The Borscht topping is dictated by personal preference. Many Russians choose to top their stew with mayonnaise rather than sour cream. They claim the salty taste of the mayo complements the sweet beet flavor of the Borscht.

Dinner

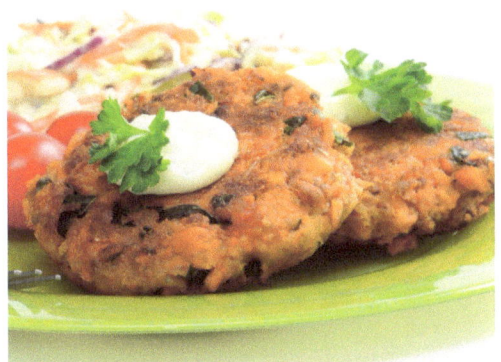

Salmon Patties

Ingredients:
- 12 ounces skinless boneless salmon
- ¼ cup white or yellow onion chopped
- ½ cup oatmeal
- ¼ cup chopped parsley, oregano, or cilantro
- 2 large eggs beaten
- 3 tbsp olive oil
- 2 tbsp real butter (preferably grassfed)
- Himalayan or sea salt
- Freshly ground black pepper

Directions:
1. In a saucepan, sauté onions in 1 tbsp oil until cooked.
2. With hands, combine salmon, onions, oatmeal, seasonings, and eggs. Form into patties.
3. Melt butter and combine with remaining oil in a pan. Brown patties for about 4-5 minutes on each side.
4. Blot excess grease and serve

Nutritional Information:
4 servings
Calories: 370
Protein: 23
Carbohydrate: 2
Fat: 28

Tips:
Serve with vegetables and rice.

Dinner

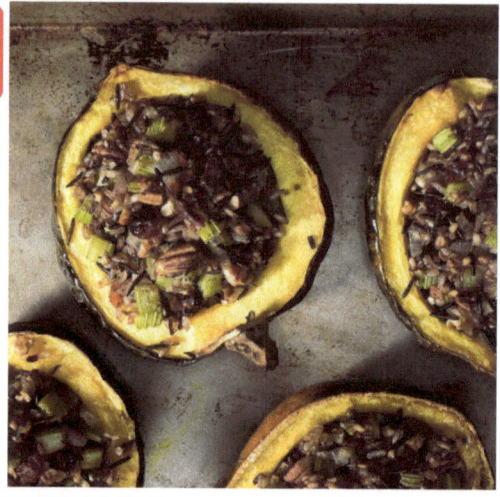

Acorn Squash

Ingredients:
- 1 acorn squash
- 3 tbsp real butter (preferably grass fed)
- 1 tsp brown sugar
- 1 tsp cinnamon
- 2 tbsp sour cream

Directions:
1. Preheat oven to 425-degrees F
2. Spread 1 tbsp butter over a baking sheet with sides
3. Cut the squash in half lengthwise. Remove the seeds. Place squash halves face down on baking sheet.
4. Bake for 20-25 minutes until golden.
5. Add a dollop of butter and sprinkle of brown sugar and cinnamon. Finish with a dollop of sour cream before serving.

Nutritional Information:
2 servings
Calories: 305.5
Protein: 2.5
Carbohydrate: 26
Fat: 20

Tips:
This makes a great light meal, a lovely side dish, or a healthy dessert.

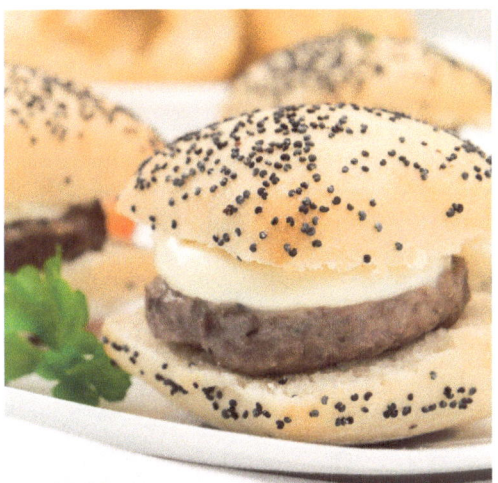

Dinner

Venison and Beef Burgers

Ingredients:
- ½ pound ground venison
- ½ pound ground 85/15% grass-fed beef
- 1 egg
- 2 tbsp Worcestershire sauce
- 2 tablespoons minced garlic
- ½ cup onion diced
- ½ green peppers diced
- Freshly ground black pepper to taste.

Directions:
1. In a large bowl, mix all ingredients. Separate into 1/3-pound patties. Use a kitchen scale for accuracy.
2. Heat a cast iron skillet and cook patties 3-4 minutes on each side, depending on desired "doneness".
3. Serve with desired toppings

Nutritional Information:
3 servings
Calories: 326
Protein: 49.7
Carbohydrate: 5.4
Fat: 15.6

Tips:
Mixing egg and ground beef reduces the dryness and gaminess that many complain about with venison.
These can also be cooked on a grill
Add cheese and mushrooms to increase protein

Dinner

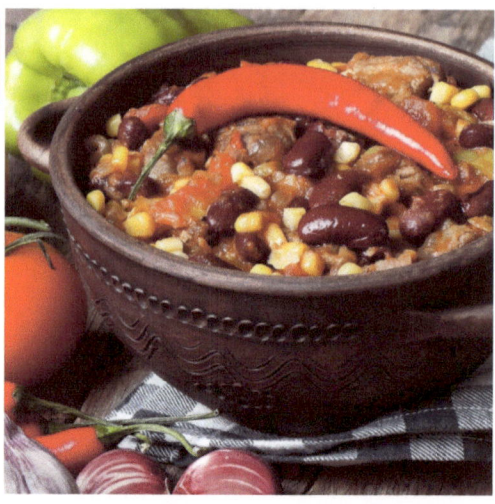

Two Meat Chili

Ingredients:
- 1 pound stew meat cut into 1-inch cubes
- 1/8 cup Worcestershire sauce
- 1 pound ground 85/15% grass-fed beef or bison
- 1 cup onion rough cut
- ½ cup green peppers (about 1 pepper)
- ½ cup red pepper (about 1 pepper)
- 2 cans chili beans
- 2 cups of chopped tomatoes (about 2 large tomatoes)
- 1 quart tomato juice
- 1 tbsp cilantro

Directions:
1. In a large skillet, brown the stew meat on medium heat with the Worcestershire sauce. Place it in a large stockpot.
2. In the same skillet, brown the ground beef or ground bison. Place it in the stockpot.
3. Add vegetables and tomato juice and bring to boil over medium heat. Then, reduce the heat to medium-low and allow to simmer for 60-120 minutes.
4. Add cilantro before serving.

Nutritional Information:
8 servings
Calories: 243
Protein: 26
Carbohydrate: 12
Fat: 10.25

Tips:
For best results cook the day before eating. The flavors combine more over time.

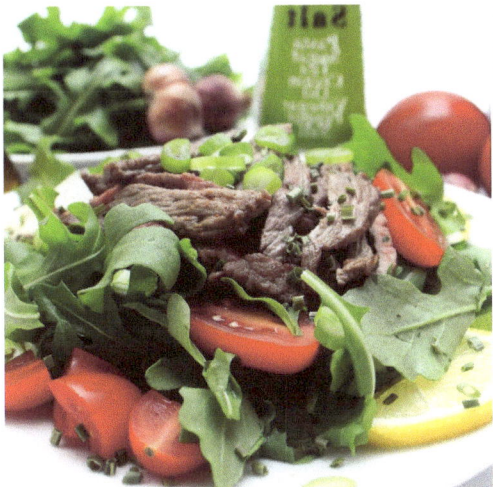

Dinner

Grilled Steak Salad

Ingredients:
- 4 4-ounce, 1 1/3-inch thick steak fillets
- 1 tsp coriander seeds
- 2 tsp freshly ground black pepper
- 2 tsp olive oil
- 4 cups kale
- 1 cup tomato cubed (about 1 medium tomato)
- 1 cucmber diced
- 2 stalks celery sliced
- ½ cup white or yellow onion diced

Directions:
1. Mix the coriander seeds and half of the pepper. Dry rub the steak fillets with the mixture. Use 1 tbsp oil to grease a large skillet and place on medium heat. Add the fillet when the skillet is warm.
2. Turn the steaks periodically and remove when it feels correct to the touch. Rare is soft, well done is firmer.
3. Let it set for 5 minutes to redistribute the juices. Cut into 1-inch pieces.
4. In a large bowl, mix kale, tomato, cucumber, celery, and onion. Add steak.
5. Top with favorite salad dressing and serve.

Nutritional Information:
4 servings
Calories: 232
Protein: 32.7   .6   .6
Carbohydrate: 5
Fat: 29

Tips:
Homemade dressings are usually tastier and healthier that manufactured. A fifty/fifty mixture of extra virgin olive oil and apple cider vinegar makes a great topper. This is a great meal when there is left over steak.

Dinner

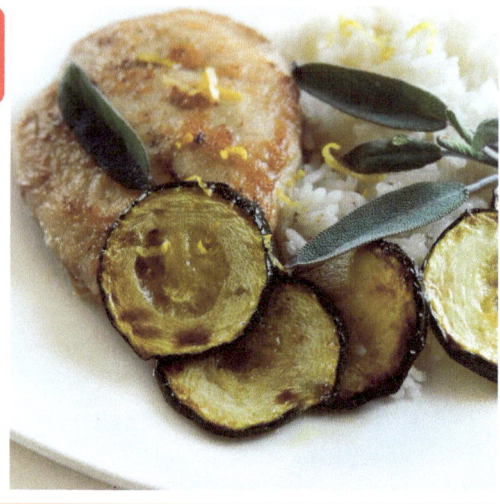

Two-Cheese Chicken and Rice Wth Zucchini

Ingredients:
- 1 tsp olive oil
- 2 pounded chicken breasts
- 2 tbsp Worcestershire sauce
- 1 soy sauce (low sodium preferably)
- ½ tsp orange zest
- 1 tsp garlic powder
- 2 cups water
- 1 cup brown rice
- 1 cup zucchini (about 1 ½ medium zucchinis)
- 2 ounces cheddar cheese shredded
- 2 ounces parmesan cheese

Directions:
1. Heat a skillet oiled with olive oil to a medium to medium-high heat. Cook for a few minutes on each side to brown. Let cook until a fork inserted in the center produces no blood. Remove from heat and cool for about 10 minutes. Cut into bite-sized pieces.
2. Place rice in a pot of water over medium heat. Bring to a boil, then reduce the heat to medium low. Cover the pot and allow to simmer for about 40 or until water is absorbed and rice is tender.
3. Add zucchini and cheese and let it sit for 10 minutes or until cheese has melted. Add chicken and stir.
4. Fluff and serve

Nutritional Information:
4 servings
Calories: 341
Protein: 35.35
Carbohydrate: 15
Fat: 14.5

Tips:
Refrigerate leftovers in an airtight container for a quick and easy lunch. Microwave at 100-percent for about 2 minutes.

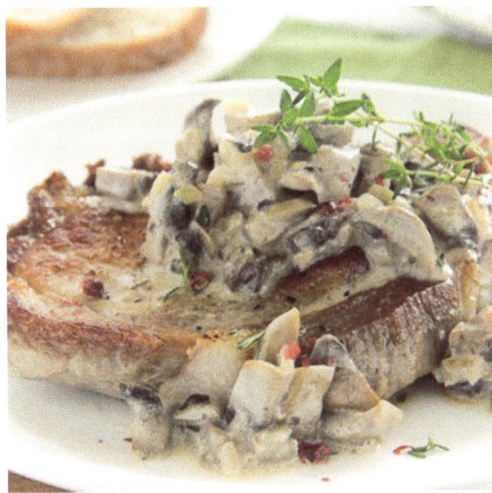

Dinner

Creamy Mushroom Pork Chops

Ingredients:
- 1 tsp olive oil
- 2/3 cup white or yellow onion (about 1 medium)
- 2 tsp minced garlic
- 4 pork-chops
- 1 10 ¾ ounce can of condensed cream of mushroom soup
- ½ cup whole milk
- 2/3 cup mushrooms sliced

Directions:
1. Heat oil in a skillet over medium-high heat. Add onions and garlic and cook until translucent.
2. Add pork-chops and cook for 4-6 minutes on each side. Continue to stir the onions and garlic.
3. In a medium sized bowl, mix the soup and milk. Add the mushrooms. Pour over the pork-chops and stir well.
4. Reduce heat and simmer for 10-15 minutes to cook pork-chops through.
5. Season and serve with vegetables and rice or mashed potatoes

Nutritional Information:
4 servings
Calories: 335
Protein: 25.7
Carbohydrate: 9.5
Fat: 30

Tips:
To ensure pork-chops are thoroughly cooked, insert an instant-read thermometer into the center. The temperature should be at least 145-degrees F.

Dinner

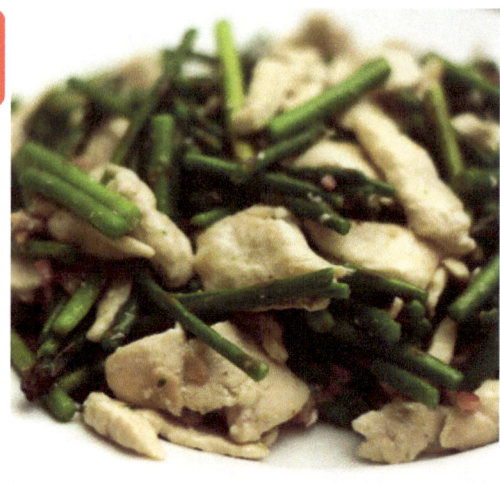

Coconut Fried Chicken With Asparagus

Ingredients:
- 1 3-pound chicken cut into 8 pieces (2 legs, 2 thighs, 2 breasts, 2 wings)
- 2 large eggs
- 1 cup flour
- 1 tsp paprika
- Himalayan or sea salt
- Freshly ground black pepper
- 1 quart coconut oil
- 2 cups asparagus (about 2 bunches)
- 1 tsp lemon juice
- 1 tsp olive oil

Directions:
1. Crack the eggs into a large bowl and beat thoroughly. Mix the salt, pepper, and paprika into the flour in a second bowl. Roll each piece of chicken first in the eggs and then in the flour.
2. Melt coconut oil in a large skillet to make about ¾-inch of oil in pan. Heat to medium or medium-high. Add chicken, cover, and fry for 15-20 minutes, turning once about half way through. Remove and use paper towels to blot up extra grease.
3. Wash asparagus and trim ends. Cut into bite-sized pieces or leave intact.
4. Fill a pot with 1-inch water. Lay asparagus in steamer basket, put inside pot, and cover. Cook on medium-high heat for 3 minutes or until asparagus is tender.
5. Remove asparagus and toss with vinegar and oil.
6. Serve hot

Nutritional Information:
4 servings
Calories: 349
Protein: 39
Carbohydrate: 2.65
Fat: 23

Tips:
If you don't have a steamer basket, either cook in a pot with very little water or microwave it wrapped in a damp paper towel for 3 minutes.

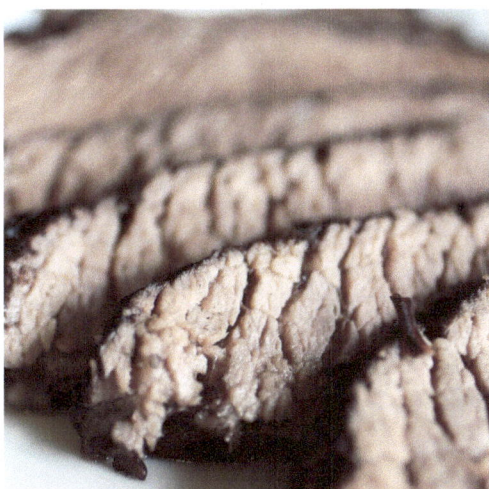

Dinner

Brisket

Ingredients:
- 3 pound fresh beef brisket
- 2 tbsp Worcestershire sauce
- 2 tbsp red wine
- 1 tbsp minced garlic
- 2 cups beef broth
- 1 cup water
- 1 tsp Himalayan or sea salt
- 1 tsp freshly ground black pepper

Directions:
1. Preheat oven to 325-degrees F
2. Trim all but 1/8-inch of fat from the meat. Place brisket in a 13x9-inch baking pan. Add all other ingredients to the meat. Cover pan with foil.
3. Bake for about 3 hours or until tender. Turn once around halfway through. Remove from heat.
4. Slice and serve with vegetables

Nutritional Information:
8 servings
Calories: 289
Protein: 37.75
Carbohydrate: 1
Fat: 14

Tips:
Cook it the night before serving to ensure maximum flavor.

Dinner

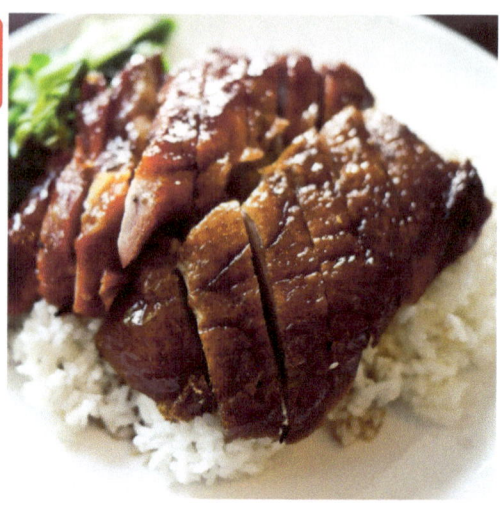

Roasted Duck

Ingredients:
- 2 5-pound ducks with insides and wing tips removed
- 1 tsp Himalayan or sea salt
- 1 tsp freshly ground pepper
- 1 tsp paprika
- 1 cup chicken broth
- ¼ cup real butter (preferably grass fed)

Directions:
1. Preheat oven to 300-degrees F
2. Prick the skin of the ducks in multiple places. Rub salt, pepper, and paprika into the skin
3. Place chicken broth and butter in a large roasting pan. Place the ducks in the pan and into the oven. Every hour, remove the ducks to prick the skin and spoon the liquid over them. Roast for 3 hours.
4. Remove the pan and drain the liquid and fat. Return the pan to the oven. Increase the temperature to 450-degree F and crisp for 30 minutes.
5. Let it rest for 10 minutes before carving and serving

Nutritional Information:
4 servings
Calories: 144
Protein: 14
Carbohydrate: 1
Fat: 8

Tips:
If desired, orange zest can be placed within the ducks to make them more aromatic.

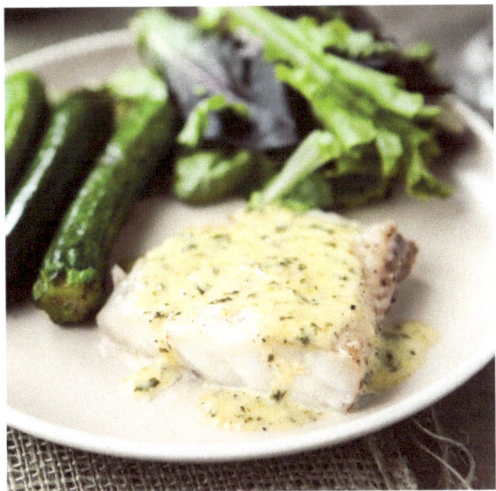

Dinner

Lemon Butter White Fish

Ingredients:
- ½ cup real butter (preferably grass fed)
- 2 tbsp fresh lemon juice
- 1 tsp Himalayan or sea salt
- 1 tsp freshly ground black pepper
- 1 tsp fresh parsley or ½ tsp dried
- 1 tbsp minced garlic
- 6 4-ounce whitefish fillets
- 2 tbsp lemon pepper

Directions:
1. Preheat oven to 350-degrees F
2. In a medium pan, melt butter and mix in lemon juice, salt, pepper, parsley, and garlic. Bring it to a boil and cook for around 10 minutes, periodically stirring.
3. Place fish on a baking sheet and cover with mixture. Add lemon pepper, cover with foil and bake 15-20 minutes or until fish is flaky.
4. Add remaining mixture and serve.

Nutritional Information:
6 servings
Calories: 370
Protein: 6
Carbohydrate: 2
Fat: 18

Tips:
This recipe can be made with cod, tilapia, or whiting.

LUNCH

Lunch

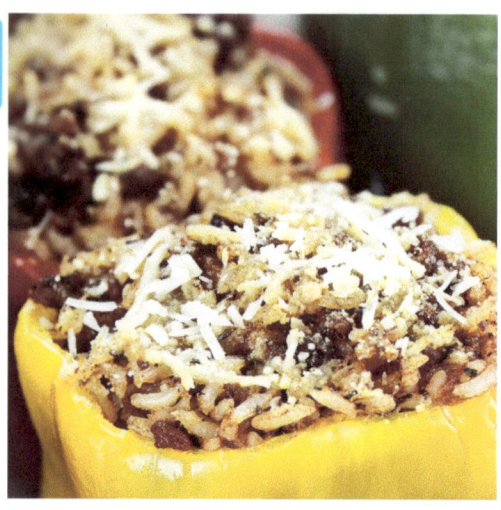

Green Pepper Stuffed With Ground Beef and Cheese

Ingredients:
- 6 green bell peppers
- Himalayan or sea salt
- 1 pound ground 85/15% beef (preferably grass fed)
- 1/3 cup white or yellow onion chopped
- freshly ground black pepper
- 1 (14 ½ ounce) can diced tomatoes
- 1 tsp Worcestershire sauce
- ½ brown rice
- 1 cup cheddar cheese shredded

Directions:
1. Cut tops from green peppers and remove seeds. Chop part of the tops to create ¼ cup.
2. Bring a pot of water to boil and add peppers. Cook for 5 minutes, then drain peppers ensuring all water is removed. Sprinkle interiors with salt.
3. In a skillet, cook beef, ¼ cup green pepper, and onion until meat is browned. Drain excess grease and return to heat. Add rice, tomatoes, Worcestershire sauce, salt and pepper. Cover and simmer for 15 minutes or until rice is tender. Remove from heat and stir in cheese until melted.
4. Preheat oven to 350-degrees F
5. Stuff peppers with the beef and rice mixture and place open-side up in a baking dish. Bake for 30 minutes or until cheese is melted and bubbly.

Nutritional Information:
6 servings
Calories: 282
Protein: 22
Carbohydrate: 17
Fat: 15

Tips:
Use spicy rotel for variety. Substitute the rice with corn and chili beans for a Mexican flavor

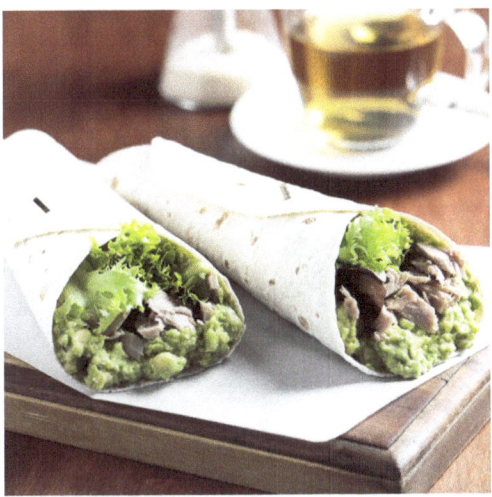

Lunch

Tuna and Avocado Wrap

Ingredients:
- ½ avocado
- ½ tsp fresh lemon juice
- 4 leaves lettuce or Swiss chard
- 2 spinach flour tortillas
- 1 can (4.5 oz.) tuna

Directions:
1. Cut the avocado in half. Store the unused half in a Ziploc bag. Use a spoon to dig the avocado fruit from the skin. Mash with a fork and add lemon juice.
2. Wash lettuce and pat dry. Place the tortillas on two plates.
3. Spread ½ avocado mixture on each tortilla. Top with 2 leaves of lettuce each.
4. Spread 1/2 can tuna on top of lettuce.
5. Wrap tightly and serve

Nutritional Information:
2 servings
Calories: 230
Protein: 13
Carbohydrate: 24
Fat: 8.5

Tips:
To ensure the remaining avocado half remains fresh longer, leave the pit in it. To keep the open side from turning brown, sprinkle a bit of lemon juice over it.

Lunch

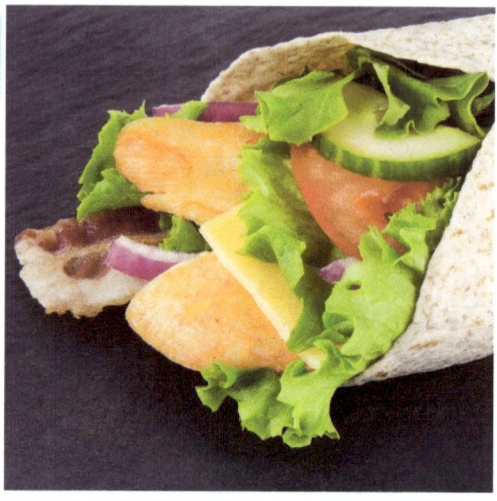

BELT

Ingredients:
- 4 slices turkey bacon
- 4 large eggs (preferably free-range)
- 1 tsp Himalayan or sea salt
- 1 tsp freshly ground black pepper
- 2 spinach flour tortillas
- 4 leaves lettuce or Swiss chard
- 2 medium tomatoes sliced

Directions:
1. Cook bacon in a skillet over medium-high heat until done to taste. Turn at least once while cooking. Remove from heat and blot excess grease.
2. In the same skillet break the eggs and rough scramble while they are cooking until done to taste. Add salt and pepper while mixing.
3. Place the tortilla on two plates. Cover each with two leaves of lettuce. Divide tomato evenly and place over lettuce. Add two slice of bacon each. Split the eggs evenly between the two servings.
4. Wrap tightly and serve.

Nutritional Information:
2 servings
Calories: 504
Protein: 18
Carbohydrate: 43.7
Fat: 14.7

Tips:
For variety, replace turkey bacon with Canadian bacon or add 2 ounces of cheese to the eggs.

Lunch

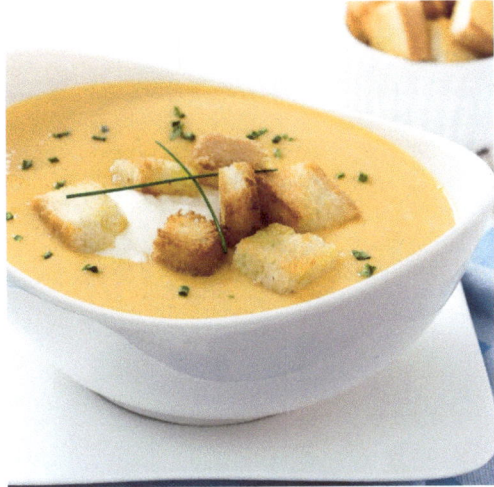

Pumpkin Soup

Ingredients:
- 1 tbsp olive oil
- 1 jalapeno pepper diced
- 1 1/2 cup fresh pureed pumpkin
- 4 cups of chicken or vegetable broth
- 1 tbsp cilantro
- 1 tbsp maple syrup

Directions:
1. Saute diced pepper in the oil in a large pot over high heat for one minute.
2. Reduce heat to medium. Add pumpkin and both. Bring to a boil and reduce heat to low. Cook for 20 minutes.
3. Add cilantro. Cook for 1 minute. Add maple syrup before serving.

Nutritional Information:
4 servings
Calories: 273
Protein: 8
Carbohydrate: 11
Fat: 7.5

Tips:
For speed and ease, replace pureed pumpkin with one can of pumpkin.

Lunch

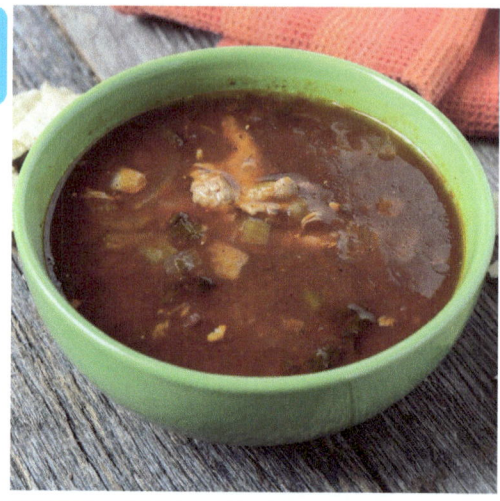

Cheesy Chicken Tortilla Soup

Ingredients:
- 1 tbsp olive oil
- 1 pound boneless chicken breast cooked and diced
- ½ cup white or yellow onion chopped
- 2 ½ cups jack cheese shredded
- ½ cup cheddar cheese shredded
- 1 ½ cups half and half
- 1 can (10 ½ ounce) cream of chicken soup (low sodium preferably)
- 2 ¾ cups whole milk
- 1/3 cup canned diced tomatoes with chilies
- 1 cup corn (canned or frozen)
- 1 can (10 ½ ounce) chili beans

Directions:
1. In oil, cook chicken on medium-high heat in a large skillet until no longer pink, dice, and set aside.
2. In a large saucepan, sauté onion. Then melt jack and cheddar cheese until melted. Stir in cream of chicken soup, and milk. Bring to a boil.
3. Add the tomatoes, corn, and beans.
4. Stir in half and half and chicken; heat through (do not boil).

Nutritional Information:
8 servings
Calories: 488
Protein: 26.5
Carbohydrate: 33.5
Fat: 7

Tips:
Serve with tortilla chips, a dollop of sour cream and avocado slices.

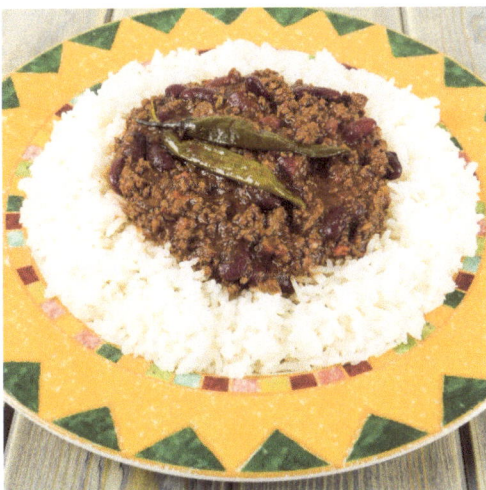

Lunch

Classic Red Beans and Rice

Ingredients:
- 1 tbsp olive oil
- 2 tbsp minced garlic
- ½ cup red onion (about 1 large) diced
- 2 stalks celery diced
- 1 green bell pepper diced
- 2 (16 ounce) cans red kidney beans
- 1 tbsp white or yellow onion diced
- 1 tsp Himalayan or sea salt
- 1/4 tsp freshly ground black pepper
- 1 tsp cayenne pepper
- 2 1/2 cups chicken broth
- 1 cup brown rice
- 1 tbsp real butter (preferably grass fed)
- 1 tbsp fresh cilantro leaves or ½ tbsp. dried

Directions:
1. Over medium-high heat, in a large saucepan, cook garlic, onion, celery, and pepper until done. Add kidney beans, diced onion, salt, and pepper. Decrease heat to low. Let beans simmer.
2. Boil chicken broth and stir in rice and butter. Bring back to a boil, then reduce heat, cover, and cook for about 20 minutes.
3. Remove from heat and let sit for about 5 minutes.
4. Gently mix rice and beans together. Serve with cilantro.

Nutritional Information:
3 servings
Calories: 405
Protein: 27
Carbohydrate: 81
Fat: 10

Tips:
Red beans and rice are a "go to" meal often used by athletes for ultimate energy when time is of the essence.

Lunch

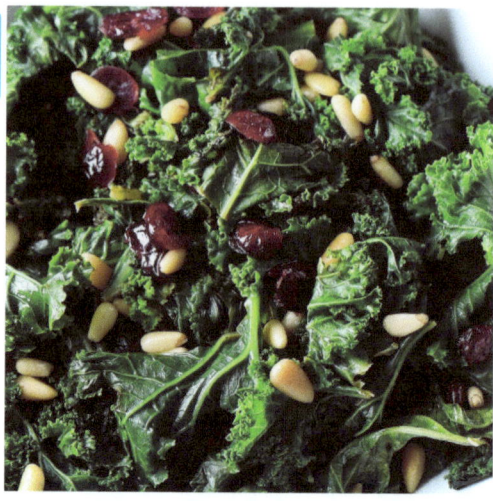

Power Salad with Kale and Nuts

Ingredients:
- 1 cup kale chopped
- 1 cup tomato chopped (about 1 medium)
- 2 stalks celery chopped
- 1 cup cucumber (about 1 medium)
- 2 tbsp raisins
- 2 tbsp almond slices
- 2 tbsp walnuts chopped
- 1 tbsp pumpkin seeds
- 1tsp chia seeds

Directions:
1. Wash all produce before chopping.
2. Combine all ingredients into a large bowl and thoroughly mix together.
3. Divide into two smaller serving bowl and top with 2-tbsp of favorite dressing.

Nutritional Information:
2 servings
Calories: 308
Protein: 9.35
Carbohydrate: 19.46
Fat: 19

Tips:
Soak all produce in cold water with ½ cup of white vinegar for ease in cleaning. This also removes any pesticide and wax from fruits and vegetables.

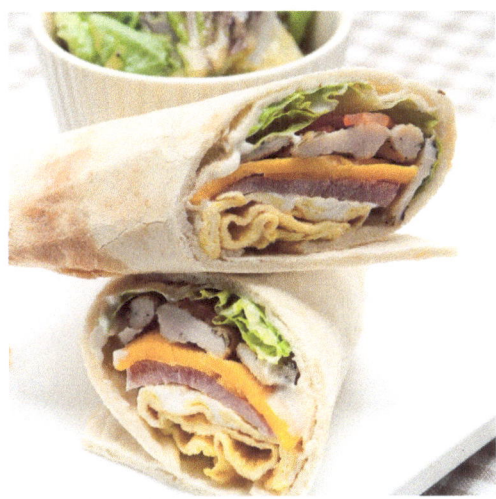

Lunch

Turkey and Bacon Wrap

Ingredients:
- 4 slices turkey bacon
- 2 spinach flour tortillas
- 2 tsp real mayonnaise
- 4 leafs lettuce or Swiss chard
- 6 ounces sliced turkey
- 2 slices Swiss cheese

Directions:
1. Cook bacon in a skillet over medium-high heat until crisp turning once half way through. Remove from heat and blot off extra fat and oil with a paper towel.
2. Place tortillas on two plates. Spread mayo evenly divided between the two.
3. Place 2 leafs of lettuce on each tortilla. Add 3 ounces of turkey to each. Place a slice of Swiss cheese on each.
4. Wrap tightly and serve.

Nutritional Information:
2 servings
Calories: 533
Protein: 61
Carbohydrate: 46
Fat: 22.2

Tips:
Although turkey has a bad "wrap" for causing drowsiness due to the tryptophan, it is very good for relieving anxiety because of its calming properties.

Lunch

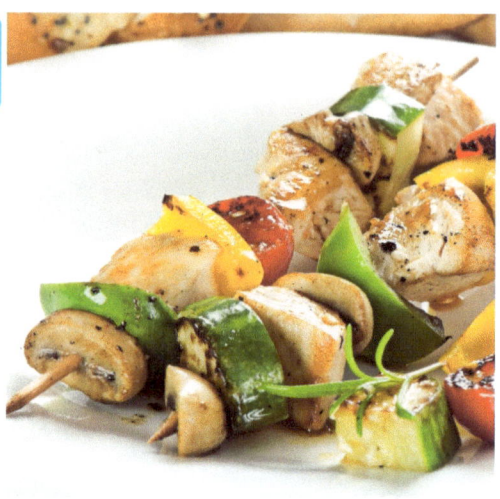

Kabob

Ingredients:
- 1/3 olive oil
- 1 tbsp Dijon mustard
- 1 tbsp Worcestershire sauce
- 1 tbsp minced garlic
- 1 tsp paprika
- 1 tsp Himalayan or sea salt
- 1 tsp freshly ground black pepper
- 1 ½ pounds lean beef cut into 1-inch cubes
- 1 large onion cut into 1-inch pieces
- 1 green pepper cut into 1-inch pieces
- 1 red pepper cut into 1-inch pieces
- 16 cap mushrooms

Directions:
1. Whisk olive oil, mustard, Worcestershire sauce, garlic, paprika, salt, and black pepper. Place in a bag. Add the beef. Seal and shake the bag. Marinate in the refrigerator at least 8 hours.
2. Place the mushrooms in the bag. Refrigerate another 8 hours.
3. Preheat grill to high heat, and oil the grate. Skewer beef, bell peppers, mushrooms, and onions skewers
4. Cook until nicely browned, turning periodically, about 15 minutes

Nutritional Information:
4 servings
Calories: 394
Protein: 35
Carbohydrate: 2.8
Fat: 25.2

Tips:
Depending on the ingredients, kabobs can be very filling and very nutritious.

Lunch

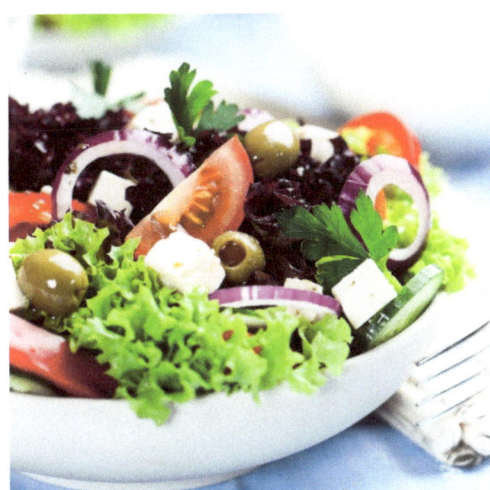

Greek Salad

Ingredients:
- 1 head Romaine lettuce torn or chopped into bite-sized pieces
- 1 medium red onion cut into thin rings
- 1 small green pepper, chopped
- 1 small red pepper, chopped
- 2 large tomatoes, chopped
- 1 medium cucumber, sliced or chopped
- ¾ cup pitted black olives (about 6 ounces)
- 1 cup feta cheese crumbles
- 6 tbsp virgin olive oil
- 1 ½ tbsp lemon juice
- 1 tbsp apple cider vinegar
- 1 tbsp minced garlic
- 1 tsp oregano
- 6 pepperoncinis
- freshly ground black pepper

Directions:
1. Combine Romaine, onion, green and red peppers, tomatoes, cucumber, olives, and cheese.
2. Whisk olive oil, lemon juice, vinegar, garlic, and oregano together until blended. Pour over salad and toss to mix.
3. Serve garnished with pepperoncinis and black pepper.

Nutritional Information:
6 servings
Calories: 252
Protein: 5.4
Carbohydrate: 9.8
Fat: 21

Tips:
Soak onion slices in a bowl of ice water for 10 minutes. This reduces the sharpness of the onion.

Lunch

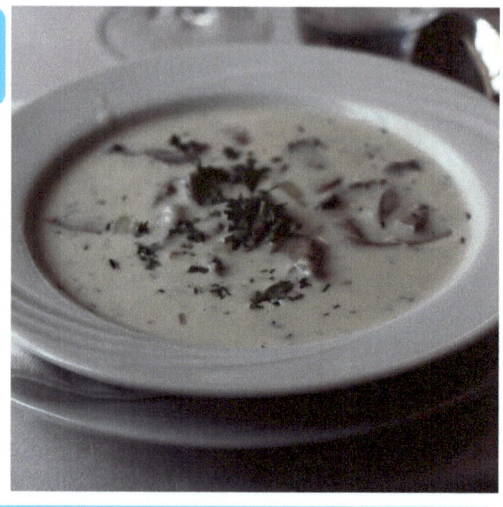

Creamy Mushrom Soup

Ingredients:
- 2 cups fresh mushroom (about 8 ounces)
- 2 tbsp white or yellow onions chopped
- 1 tbsp minced garlic
- 2 tbsp butter
- 3 tbsp all purpose flour
- 2 cups chicken or vegetable broth
- 1 cup whole milk or light cream
- ½ tsp nutmeg
- ½ tsp Himalayan or sea salt
- ½ freshly ground black pepper

Directions:
1. Cut the mushrooms into chunks. Chop onion.
2. In a large pan, melt butter and add mushrooms, onion, and garlic. Cook until they're soft. Stir in 2 tbsp flour and broth.
3. Cook until thickened, stirring periodically. Add cream and last tbsp. flour. Add nutmeg, salt, and pepper and heat until thick. Stir often and serve.

Nutritional Information:
4 servings
Calories: 333
Protein: 7.8
Carbohydrate: 9.6
Fat: 8.25

Tips:
The longer the soup simmers, the thicker it will be.

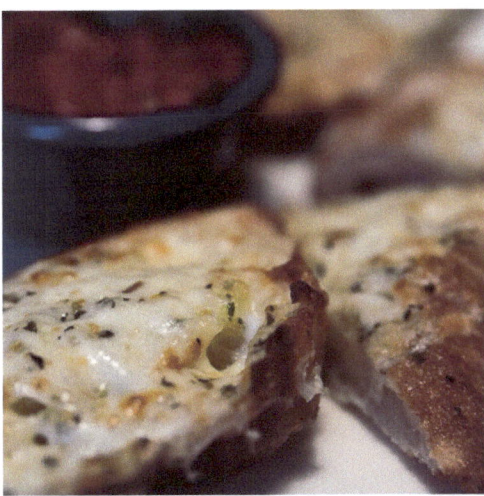

Lunch

Cheesy Bread with Tomato

Ingredients:
- 1 loaf of Italian or French bread
- 1 stick real butter melted
- 1 tbsp minced garlic
- 1-2 tsp fresh parsley or oregano finely chopped
- 2 medium tomatoes thinly sliced
- 1/3 cup mozzarella cheese shredded
- 1/3 cup parmesan cheese shredded
- 1/3 cup Romano cheese shredded

Directions:
1 Preheat oven to 400-degrees F.
2. Slice the bread lengthwise. Slice the tomatoes. Stir garlic and parsley or oregano into the melted butter. Spread over the two halves of bread.
3. Cover with tinfoil with the open sides of the bread together and bake for 15 minutes.
4. Remove from oven and open the bread. Add the tomato slices and spread the cheese evenly over the tomatoes on the open sides of the bread. Leave the bread with the cheesy side up and return to oven for another 4-5 minutes or until cheese melts.

Nutritional Information:
4 servings
Calories: 674
Protein: 22
Carbohydrate: 61
Fat: 70

Tips:
To substitute dried ingredients, use 3/4 tsp garlic and 1/2-1 tsp dried parsley or oregano.

Lunch

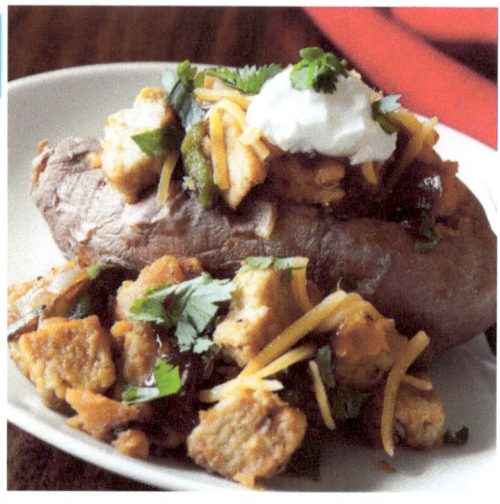

Loaded Baked Potato

Ingredients:
- 1 brown potato medium
- 2 slices turkey bacon
- ¼ cup steamed broccoli
- ¼ cup grated cheddar cheese
- 1 tsp melted butter
- 1 tsp sour cream
- 1 tsp chives

Directions:
1. Preheat oven to 425-degree F. Thoroughly wash potato, then rub it with olive oil and sprinkle it with salt.
2. Place the potato directly on the center rack or on a cookie sheet on the center rack. Bake for 45-60 minutes until a fork can be easily inserted into the center.
3. Allow to cool for 5 minutes. Cut lengthwise
4. In a skillet, cook bacon over medium heat, flipping it periodically until crisp. Remove from heat and blot grease and crumble into ½ pieces.
5. Top potato halves with broccoli, bacon, cheese, butter, sour cream, and chives

Nutritional Information:
1 servings
Calories: 559
Protein: 19.3
Carbohydrate: 38
Fat: 32.7

Tips:
For a faster potato cooking time, microwave it. Just cook at 100-percent for 5 minutes. Turn it over and cook for another 3-5 minutes until a fork can be easily inserted into the center.

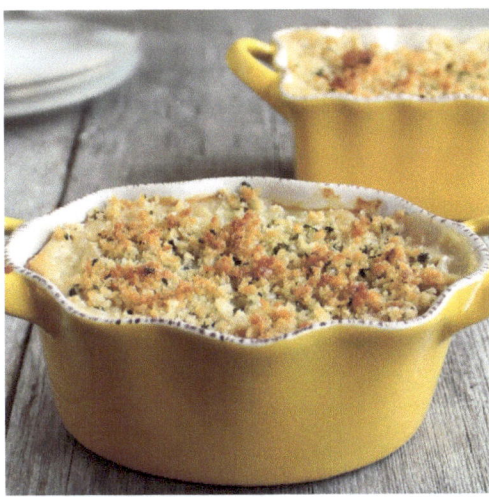

Lunch

Cheesy Quinoa

Ingredients:
- 8 slices turkey bacon crumbled
- 2 cups broccoli chopped
- 1 ¾ cups vegetable or chicken broth
- 1 cup quinoa
- 1 cup cheddar cheese (about 4 ounces) shredded
- Himalayan or sea salt
- Freshly ground black pepper

Directions:
1. In a large skillet, cook bacon until crisp turning at least once.
2. In a medium-sized pot, mix broccoli, broth, and quinoa. Bring to boil over high heat and then reduce to medium-low and cover. Simmer 15-20 minutes or until broth had been absorbed.
3. Add cheddar cheese and allow it to melt. Stir in bacon crumbles and season with salt and pepper.

Nutritional Information:
6 servings
Calories: 212
Protein: 14
Carbohydrate: 40
Fat: 58.5

Tips:
Although this is a great lunch choice it can also be used as a side dish with dinner. Just omit the bacon.

Lunch

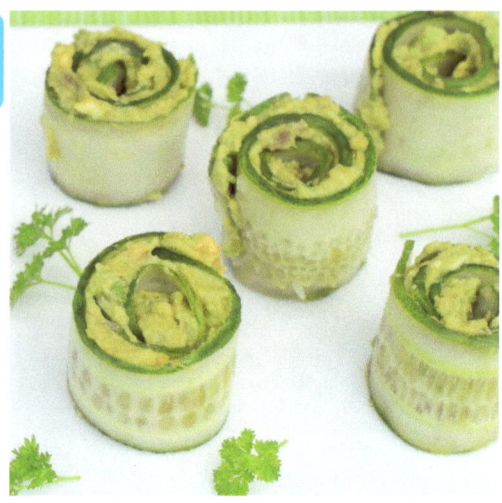

Cucumber and Avocado Roll

Ingredients:
- 1 large cucumber
- 3 avocados
- ¼ cup green onions
- ½ tsp Himalayan or sea salt
- ½ tsp freshly ground black pepper
- ¼ cup fresh parsley diced
- 1/8 cup fresh dill diced
- 2 tbsp fresh lemon juice

Directions:
1. Wash cucumbers and thin slice lengthwise.
2. Cut avocados and use a spoon to remove the fruit from the skin. Use a fork to mash and add the rest of the ingredients.
3. Spread mixture across the cucumber slices and roll. Use remaining mixture to "glue" the end.
4. Refrigerate any leftovers

Nutritional Information:
3 servings
Calories: 337
Protein: 4
Carbohydrate: 21
Fat: 30

Tips:
Turn this into sushi by rolling the rolls over cooked rice.

BREAKFAST

Breakfast

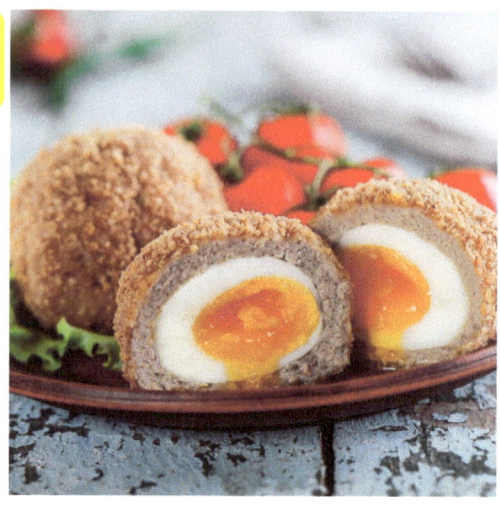

Scotch Eggs

Ingredients:
- 1 pound pork sausage
- 2 tsp Worcestershire sauce
- ½ cup cheddar cheese
- 1 tsp garlic powder
- ½ tsp Himalayan or sea salt
- ½ tsp freshly ground black pepper
- 1 large egg raw (preferably free-range)
- 6 large eggs hard cooked

Directions:
1. In a medium sized pot, boil 6 eggs for 10 minutes. Drain eggs and place in ice water to cool before peeling.
2. Preheat oven to 350-degree F
3. With your hands, mix sausage, Worcestershire sauce, cheese garlic, salt, pepper, and one egg in a medium sized bowl
4. Divide into 6 equal pieces, flatten, and wrap around the boiled eggs.
5. Arrange the on a baking sheet and bake for 30 minutes.

Nutritional Information:
6 servings
Calories: 250
Protein: 24
Carbohydrate: 0.9
Fat: 16

Tips:
Serve with a small side salad to make a larger meal. These also make great appetizers at dinner parties.

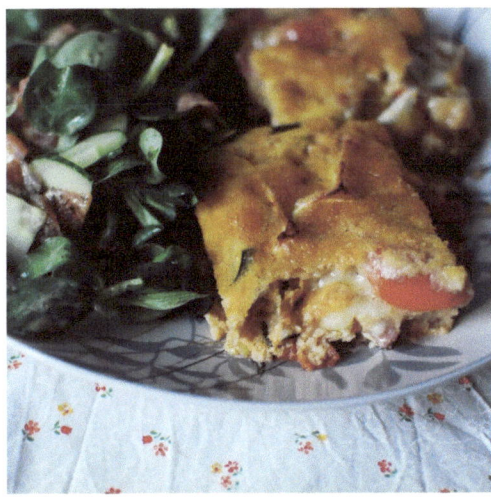

Breakfast

Bacon Egg Bake

Ingredients:
- 4 slices turkey bacon
- 1 dozen large eggs (free range preferably)
- ½ cup whole milk
- 2 ounces cheddar cheese shredded
- ½ cup onion diced
- ½ tsp Himalayan or sea salt
- ½ tsp freshly ground pepper
- ½ tsp turmeric or paprika

Directions:
1. Preheat oven to 350-degree F
2. Fry bacon in a skillet on medium heat flipping periodically until crisp. Remove bacon, blot off grease, and crumble into ½-inch sized pieces.
3. Crack eggs into a medium sized mixing bowl. Whisk briskly until thoroughly combined. Whisk in milk. Add crumbled bacon, onion, and shredded cheese. Add seasonings.
4. Pour mixture evenly into a 12-cup muffin tin that has been sprayed with nonstick olive oil spray.
5. Cook for 20-25 minutes or until a knife inserted into the middle comes out clean.

Nutritional Information:
12 servings
Calories: 113
Protein: 7.9
Carbohydrate: 1.6
Fat: 7

Tips:
Leftover servings can be frozen in Ziploc bags for a quick meal or snack throughout the week. Just microwave them for 40 seconds at 70-percent power.

Breakfast

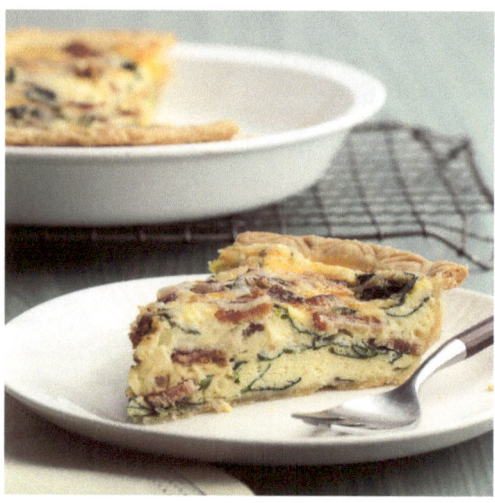

Three Cheese Bacon and Tomato Quiche

Ingredients:
- 1 9-inch frozen deep piecrust
- 3 slices turkey bacon
- ½ cup red onion
- 4 ounces Swiss cheese
- 2 ounces Parmesan cheese
- 2 ounces cheddar cheese
- 4 large eggs (preferably free range)
- 1 cup half and half

Directions:
1. Preheat oven to 375-degrees F
2. Place piecrust in a pie pan, and bake it for 10 minutes.
3. In a frying pan, cook chopped bacon and onion over medium-high heat until done. Mix the bacon, onions, and three cheeses and pour into the piecrust.
4. In a medium bowl, mix the eggs and half and half. Pour over the cheese mixture in the piecrust.
5. Add the tomatoes slices around the entire top.
6. Bake for 40 minutes or until the top begins to brown.

Nutritional Information:
8 servings
Calories: 285
Protein: 12.75
Carbohydrate: 15.6
Fat: 17.68

Tips:
The yolks of free-range eggs are usually much darker than other eggs. This is due to the additional vitamins they contain. Yellow yolks have far fewer vitamins than free-range ones.

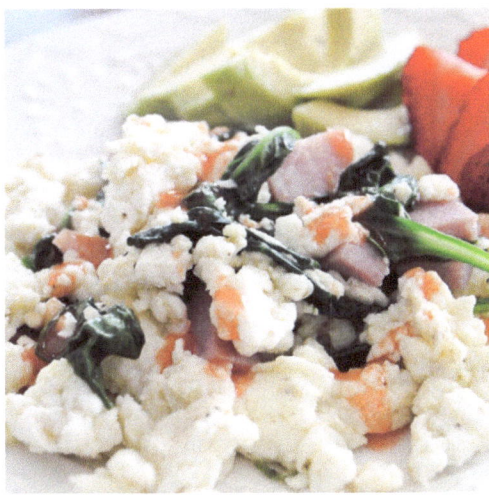

Breakfast

Mediterranean Style Egg Scramble

Ingredients:
- 8 large eggs (preferably free-range)
- 2 tbsp fresh parsley or 1 tbsp dreid
- 1 tsp fresh oregano or ½ tsp dried
- 3 tbsp green onion chopped
- freshly ground black pepper
- 1 tbsp olive oil
- 2 cups fresh spinach torn into bite sized pieces
- 1 cup feta crumbled
- 1 cup cherry tomatoes halved
- ¼ cup pitted black olives

Directions:
1. In a medium-sized bowl, break eggs and beat with a whisk. Stir in parsley, oregano, green onion, and pepper.
2. Over medium heat, place a 10-inch skillet. After 10 minutes, add olive oil and increase heat to medium-high. Add spinach and cook for about 2 ½ minutes or until wilted.
3. Add egg mixture and slowly scramble into the spinach. When eggs are nearly done, but still moist, add feta and cook until it begins to melt, then add tomatoes and olives.

Nutritional Information:
4 servings
Calories: 410
Protein: 5
Carbohydrate: 5
Fat: 8.25

Tips:
Serve with a side of avocado slices for added nutrition and flavor.

Breakfast

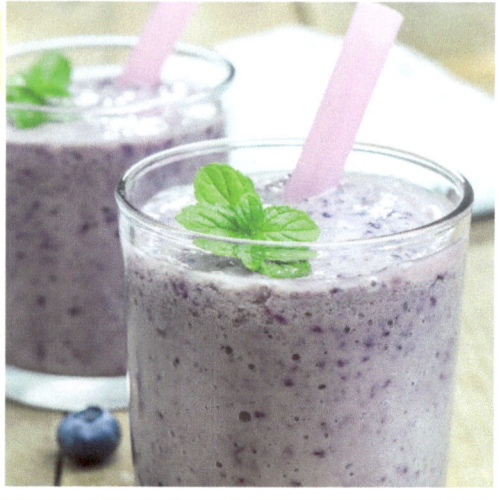

Berry Protein Smoothie

Ingredients:
- ½ cup blueberries
- ½ cup strawberries
- ½ cup grated carrot (about 1 carrot)
- 1 cup unsweetened vanilla almond milk
- 1 ½ tbsp almond butter
- 5 ice cubes

Directions:
1. Wash produce
2. Place all ingredients in a blender and mix until thoroughly combined.
3. Serve immediately

Nutritional Information:
1 serving
Calories: 300
Protein: 8.25
Carbohydrate: 36
Fat: 15

Tips:
Make a week's worth of smoothies at a time by combining all ingredients besides the ice and place in individual containers in the refrigerator. Just add ice when blending.

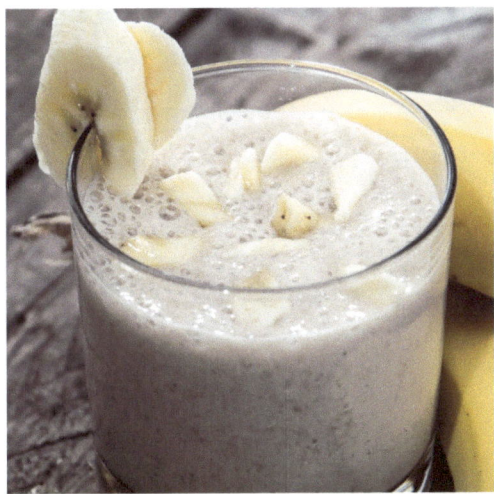

Peanut Butter Banana Smoothie

Ingredients:
- 2 bananas
- ½ cup spinach
- 1 cup unsweetened vanilla almond milk
- ½ cup peanut butter
- 5 ice cubes

Directions:
1. Wash spinach
2. Place all ingredients in a blender and mix until thoroughly combined.
3. Serve immediately

Nutritional Information:
1 serving
Calories: 554
Protein: 20
Carbohydrate: 76
Fat: 36

Tips:
Overripe bananas are healthier and more nutritious than under ripe ones. Many people find a mushy banana gross, so using them in smoothies is a great way to receive the benefits without

Breakfast

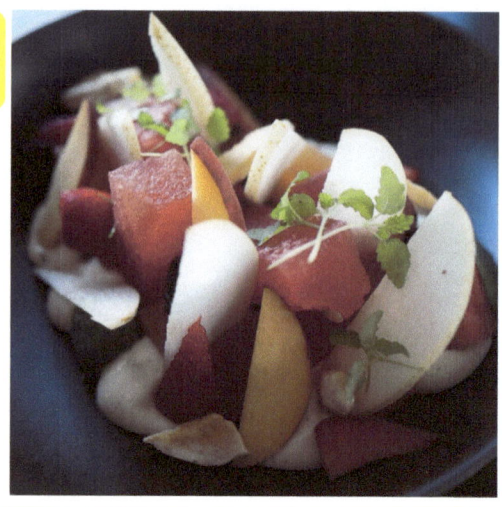

Fruit Salad with Nuts and Cheese

Ingredients:
- 1 red apple medium cored and diced
- 1 yellow apple medium cored and diced
- 1 Granny Smith apple medium
- 1 cup seedless grapes halved
- 1/3 cup almonds sliced
- 1/3 cup walnuts chopped
- 1/3 cup pecans chopped
- 1 ½ cup yogurt
- 4 ounces cheddar cheese cubed

Directions:
1. Wash the fruit thoroughly. Core and dice the apples. Halve the grapes.
2. In a large bowl, combine the apples, grapes, almonds, walnuts, and pecans. Stir to mix. Add the yogurt and stir. Fold in the cheese.
3. Refrigerate for an hour before serving

Nutritional Information:
6 servings
Calories: 340
Protein: 11
Carbohydrate: 17
Fat: 29

Tips:
To avoid browning, sprinkle the diced apples with lemon juice before mixing.

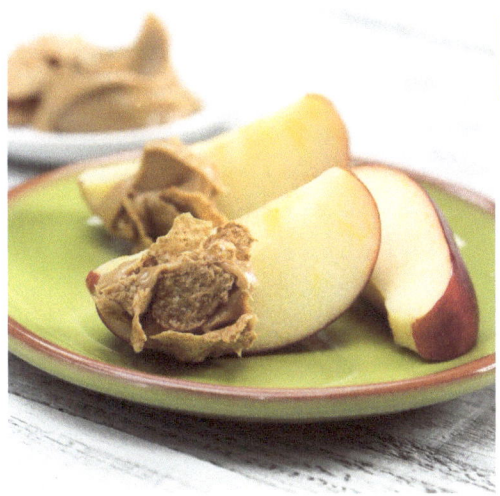

Breakfast

Apple Slices with Almond Butter

Ingredients:
- 1 red apple medium sliced
- 1 yellow apple medium sliced
- 1 Granny Smith apple medium sliced
- 4 tbsp almond butter

Directions:
1. Wash the apples and core them. Cut them into slices about 1/2-inch wide.
2. Serve with almond butter

Nutritional Information:
2 servings
Calories: 340
Protein: 5.5
Carbohydrate: 29
Fat: 11

Tips:
The almond butter can be eaten as a dip or spread over the slices to evenly distribute it.

Breakfast

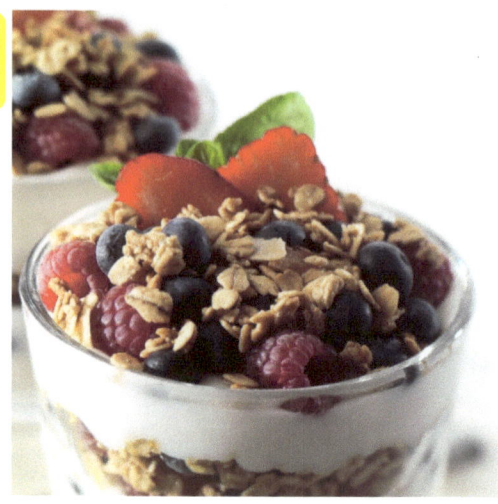

Yogurt with Nuts and Seeds

Ingredients:
- 1 cup yogurt plain
- 1 tsp honey
- 1 tbsp almonds sliced
- 1 tbsp walnuts chopped
- 1 tsp chia seeds
- 1 tsp flax seeds

Directions:
1. Stir honey into the yogurt.
2. Add almonds, walnuts, chia seeds, and flax seeds.
3. Chill for 30 minutes or serve immediately

Nutritional Information:
1 serving
Calories: 336
Protein: 13.4
Carbohydrate: 23.3
Fat: 20.3

Tips:
This is a recipe that the preparer can get creative with. For variety experiment with substituting different nuts or add fruit.

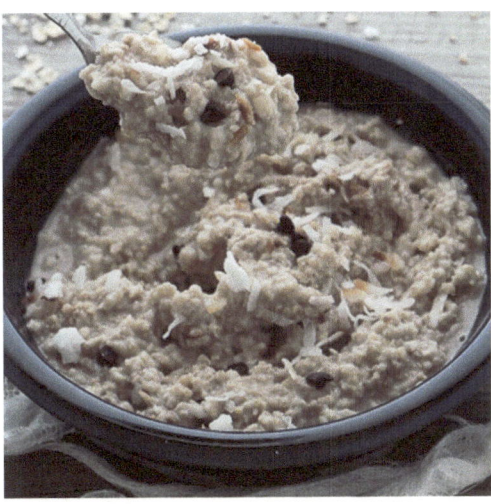

Breakfast

Cooked Oats with Coconut Oil and Nuts

Ingredients:
- 4 cups water
- 1 cup steel cut oats
- 1/8 tsp Himalayan or sea salt
- 2 tbsp coconut oil
- 2 tbsp almonds sliced
- 2 tbsp walnuts chopped
- 1 tbsp chia seeds
- 1 tbsp flax seeds

Directions:
1. Place water in a pot and bring to boil over high heat.
2. Stir in the oats and salt. Bring back to a boil stirring periodically.
3. Reduce heat to low and simmer for about 20-30 minutes, stirring periodically. The longer they cook, they thicker the oatmeal.
4. Remove from heat. Stir in the oil, almonds, walnuts, chia seeds, and flax seeds.
5. Serve after 5 minutes.

Nutritional Information:
4 servings
Calories: 151
Protein: 5
Carbohydrate: 19
Fat: 12

Tips:
Leftover oats can be kept refrigerated in an airtight container up to a week. As they will thicken, stir in a bit of milk or water before reheating.

SNACKS

Snack

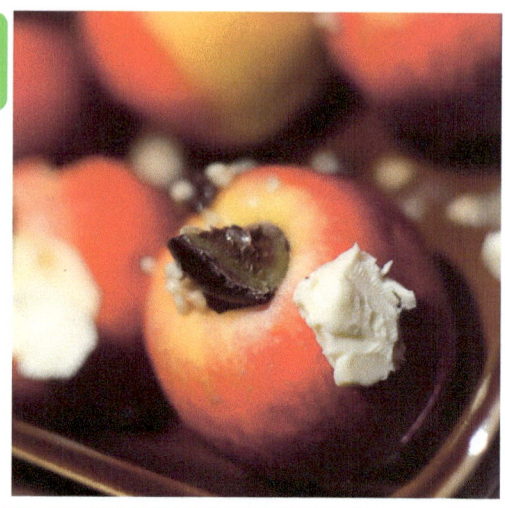

Baked Apple with Butter

Ingredients:
- 4 tart apples
- 4 tbsp butter (grassfed preferably)
- 4 tsp cinnamon
- 1 tsp nutmeg

- Directions:
1. Preheat oven to 350-degree F
2. Wash and core apples leaving the bottom intact.
3. Place 1 tbsp butter in each apple. Follow by sprinkling each with the cinnamon and nutmeg.
4. On a baking sheet, bake for 12-18 minutes.
5. Cool slightly and serve

Nutritional Information:
4 servings
Calories: 205
Protein: 1.0
Carbohydrate: 24.7
Fat: 10.3

Tips:
Consider serving ala mode with ½ cup vanilla ice cream.

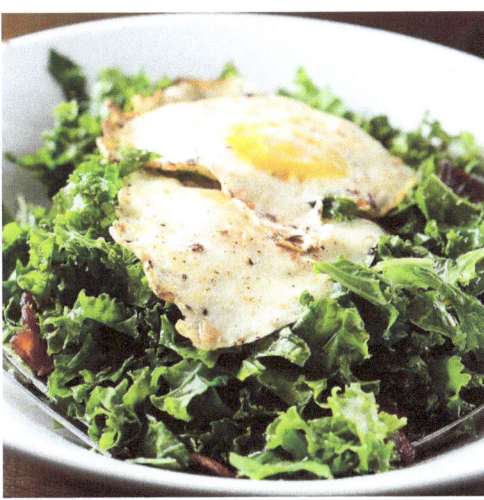

Hard Cooked Egg with Kale

Ingredients:
- 7 large eggs
- 1 tbsp Dijon mustard
- 1 cup olive oil
- 3 tsp white vinegar or lemon juice
- ½ tsp Himalayan or sea salt
- ½ freshly ground black pepper
- 3 cups kale chopped

Directions:
1. In a medium sized bowl, combine the yolk from one of the eggs and the mustard. Use a whisk to mix well. While whisking, add a thin stream of the oil until completely mixed. Whisk in the vinegar or lemon juice, salt, and pepper. Cover and refrigerate
2. Place the other 6 eggs in a large pot and cover them with water. Cook on the stovetop on high heat to a rolling boil. Time for 9 minutes then remove and immediately immerse the eggs in ice-water. Once they are cooled, peel and slice them.
3. Divide the kale into three serving bowls. Mix 1 tbsp of the homemade mixture into each. Divide the egg slices evenly between the three bowls.
4. Chill for 30 minutes or serve immediately.

Nutritional Information:
3 servings
Calories: 521
Protein: 13
Carbohydrate: 12.7
Fat: 40.5

Tips:
Eggs continue to cook after they have been removed from heat. Cooling them immediately is necessary to avoid overcooking.

Snack

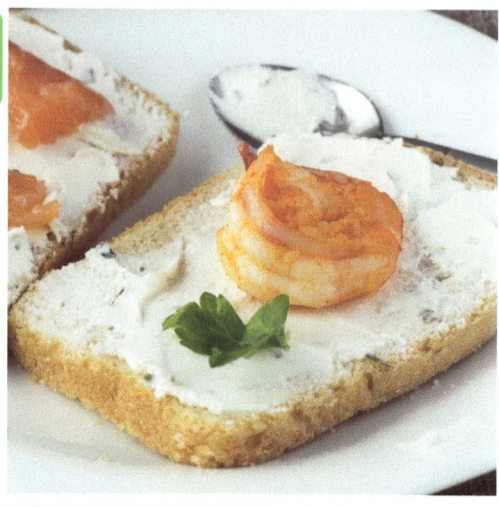

Salmon Spread with Cream Cheese

Ingredients:
- 4 ounces smoked salmon minced
- 8 ounces cream cheese
- ½ cup sour cream
- 2 tsp fresh oregano
- 2 tsp fresh cilantro
- ½ tsp Himalayan or sea salt
- ½ tsp freshly ground black pepper

Directions:
1. Mix the cream cheese and sour cream. Add the oregano, cilantro, salt, and pepper.
2. Chill for 30-60 minutes. Serve with fresh, raw vegetables, rice cakes, or rye bread.

Nutritional Information:
12 servings
Calories: 98
Protein: 3.5
Carbohydrate: 1
Fat: 9.6

Tips:
To use dry seasonings rather than fresh, substitute 1 tsp dry oregano for 2 fresh, and 1 tsp dry cilantro for 2 fresh.

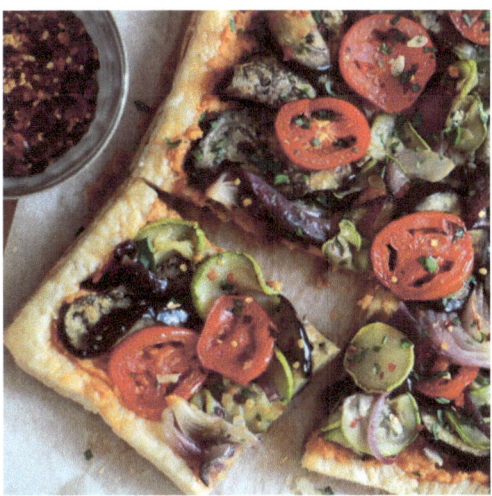

Mediterranean Veggie Plate with Hummus

Ingredients:
- 1 can garbanzo beans
- 1 tsp minced garlic (about 1 peeled clove)
- 2 tbsp fresh lemon juice
- ¼ cup roasted tahini
- ¼ cup water
- 1 tbsp extra-virgin olive oil
- ½ tsp Himalayan or sea salt
- 4 stalks celery cut into 3-inch "sticks"
- 4 carrots cut into 3-inch "sticks"
- 1 medium cucumber sliced
- 16 cherry tomatoes
- 1 green pepper sliced
- 1 red pepper sliced
- 16 pitted black olives

Directions:
1. Drain and rinse beans. Combine beans, garlic, lemon juice, tahini, water, olive oil, and salt in a food processor. Blend until smooth adding water as needed, one tbsp.
2. Place in a bowl and drizzle the olive oil over it.
3.Cut vegetables and serve

Nutritional Information:
4 servings
Calories: 75
Protein: 3
Carbohydrate: 13
Fat: 2.1

Tips:
Cover and refrigerate left over hummus. In an airtight container it will keep for 1 week.

Snack

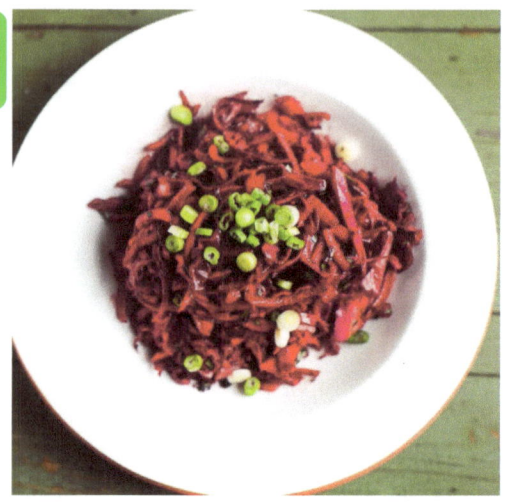

Beet and Cabbage Salad

Ingredients:
- 4 cups cabbage (about ½ head)
- 2 beets medium
- 2 carrots
- 2 stalks celery
- ½ red onion
- ¼ cup fresh parsley or 1/8 cup dried
- ¼ cup apple cider vinegar
- ¼ cup virgin olive oil
- 1 tsp Himalayan or sea salt
- ½ tsp freshly ground black pepper

Directions:
1. Wash all produce in cold water. Core the cabbage and peel the beets. Shred or chop the cabbage, beets, carrots, and celery. Chop and add onion and parsley.
2. In a small bowl, whisk vinegar, oil, salt, and pepper together.
3. Mix into the slaw and refrigerate 20-30 minutes before serving

Nutritional Information:
4 servings
Calories: 172
Protein: 2
Carbohydrate: 50
Fat: 14

Tips:
Making the day before and refrigerating overnight enhances the flavor.
This can also be made using a food processor to chop the vegetables.

In Conclusion

Basically, by eating more of a whole food based diet with a high fat content and low carb content, you can not only lose weight without feeling hungry, in return it will keep your body always using fat as it's main fuel source.

You choose meat, eggs, fish, and low-carb vegetables and avoid sugar and starches, such as bread and pasta. Try to avoid processed, factoryproduced foods. They will leave your body in an unbalanced state both mentally and physically.

Pair this with a proper training program and you will lose weight even faster. I recommend refraining from substituting sugar with harmful aspartame or other sugar-substitutes, as these may contribute to other problems including weight gain, which can also increase your cravings even more for those sugary foods.

By following this plan, weight loss can occur without having to count calories or adhering to restrictive portion sizes. Try it for yourself and enjoy!

For more inspiration visit http://www.fastfit60.com

I WOULD LOVE TO HEAR FROM YOU

Tell Me bout Your Progress

Nowadays, it is fairly common to come across empty promises made by "fitness gurus." I am a strong believer in helping people achieve their goals and guiding them to success. My mission is to reach as many people as I can by spreading information and knowledge that will inspire others to achieve their health and fitness goals. I am committed to changing people's lives, and I want you to join me.

I offer a free newsletter to many subscribers nationwide.

http://faithfulfitnesskc.com/newsletter/

Stay connected with me on my Instagram.

https://instagram.com/fastfit60/

I am passionate about helping anyone and everyone in this journey of life. Stay in contact with me and let me know how you are doing. I would love to hear how the program is working for you, what you have achieved along the way, or if you have any comments or questions. I am here to help you reach your goals- both inside and outside the gym.

Your Dedicated Coach

ALEX COFFEY

www.ingramcontent.com/pod-product-compliance
Lightning Source LLC
Chambersburg PA
CBHW050813290526
45792CB00001B/91